MEDITATIONS ON THE PRINCIPLES OF T'AI CHI

MEDITATIONS ON THE PRINCIPLES OF T'AI CHI

A Beginner's Guided Reflection to Cultivate *Your* T'ai Chi

WILLIAM DONNELLY

ISBN (print) 979-8-9879559-2-5
ISBN (epub) 979-8-9879559-3-2

Cover and Interior Book Design by Happenstance Type-O-Rama.

Published by
Apeirogon Publishing
Patchogue, New York

CONTENTS

Introduction. 1

How to Use This Book. 6

Before you Begin 7

Week One 9
Wuji: No Extremes

Week Two 17
Breath

Week Three 25
Learning and Self-Discovery Takes Time

Week Four 35
Yin Yang: Integrated Opposites

Week Five 45
Settle the Qi

Week Six 53
Intention

Week Seven 61
Your Center

Week Eight 71
Rooting

Week Nine 79
Alignment

Week Ten 87
Meditation + Qi Gong = T'ai Chi

Week Eleven 95
Principle or Sequence—Where Is the Focus?

Week Twelve 105
Your T'ai Chi Path

Final Thoughts 115

Acknowledgments 117
About the Author 118

INTRODUCTION

T'ai Chi is practiced by over four million people globally and the numbers are growing. The benefits have been the subject of several books, including one by Harvard Medical School researcher Peter M. Wayne, PhD. T'ai Chi is often depicted in Hollywood films as the highest level of martial arts training, appearing in movies like *Road House, The Recruit,* and *Lethal Weapon.* Corporate executives and celebrities are increasingly embracing this art. There has been a gradual, persistent wave of recognition that T'ai Chi is not just for the aging, but rather a transformative path to a higher quality of life for anyone.

T'ai Chi is a four-thousand-year-old art that encompasses a philosophy, a system of health, and a method of self-defense. Its underlying philosophy, Taoism, is best described as a philosophy of nature. Qi Gong, its health system, is known as the science of nature. These two combined form the basis of strategy and power in T'ai Chi's self-defense applications. Understanding this progression is essential to fully understanding your T'ai Chi lessons and practice.

To begin the process, you must first learn to calm the mind through meditation. Then you need to understand the pluralistic philosophy of Taoism, which underpins the Qi Gong exercises and the entire T'ai Chi form. Qi Gong exercises maintain the meditative state while developing the internal physical structure, which enables you to discover your intrinsic energy. These three elements—meditation, Taoism, and Qi Gong—establish the foundation by which you can discover an ideal mental and physical state. From here you learn T'ai Chi techniques, form, and eventually martial applications. This process is your gateway to a lifetime of discovery, reflection, cultivation, and refinement.

Self-discovery is the illumination of truth—your true self, which is revealed through continued practice. Self-discovery reveals your purpose, personal power, and capacity to act. You discover the meaning of your life.

As your awareness increases, it is equally important to reflect on what you are learning and the purpose it has in your life. Reviewing, contemplating, and writing about your weekly lessons and discoveries will help you understand and apply the principles of T'ai Chi. You are documenting an awareness of your new path of living.

Reflecting on your experience will also create a more meaningful transformation. You will naturally have more questions, which lead to greater understanding. Reflection will bring clarity and purpose to your practice.

Once you discover and reflect, you must cultivate your knowledge through experience. You put your learning into practice. This is where you seek to develop and improve on what you have learned. Through your work on the physical elements of T'ai Chi, you will internalize its core principles. Like a tree, you are establishing your roots so that you can later grow branches.

You refine what you learn by continuously seeking to remove what is nonessential in thought and movement. Through learning, practice, and introspection, you strip away the meaningless self-perceptions and attitudes, labels, and concepts that preoccupy you. As you reduce the outside noise, you are left with only that which is vital. This is when you will experience your self-discoveries. Then the cycle of self-discovery, reflection, cultivation, and refinement begins again. It is an endlessly fascinating process, and this book is here to guide your start.

Why I Wrote This Book

Over my twenty-five years of teaching, I have noticed that some beginner students intuitively understand T'ai Chi, while others come to this understanding as an epiphany a few months later. T'ai Chi is a very deep and subtle art that can be difficult to comprehend during the early training stages. Teaching styles and emphases vary, but whether you begin with fundamental Qi Gong, stance work, and hand techniques or dive right into the T'ai Chi form, understanding and integrating the foundational principles early is key to long-term quality. However, the principles and purpose can seem obscure to a new student.

My own teaching approach focuses the student on the fundamental elements before bringing them together in the T'ai Chi form. The students embrace the lessons, but sometimes admit later that they didn't have a clear sense of what we were doing or where we were headed in those early stages.

This realization—that, to the novice, the early lessons often seem unclear and unrelated—inspired me to write this book, in which I have set out to identify and communicate one essential element of T'ai Chi every week. Each element exists everywhere in T'ai Chi training, so it does not need to be aligned with a specific technique or form. My intention is to raise your awareness of a principle so that you can reflect on its physical, mental/philosophical, and even spiritual impact. Then, you can more fully apply the principles into other parts of your life. The principles will gradually become more holistic—vital elements of existence and in how you interact with the world around you.

By integrating the T'ai Chi principles into our lives, we bring them to life. We live the life of T'ai Chi ("grand ultimate").

An Open-Minded Approach to Your Learning

Though many people seem to be in a rush to finish things these days, the true beauty and wonder of learning T'ai Chi is right now: the point where you are entering this practice as a beginner. You are curious and have questions. This is a good thing! The questioning mind—the beginner's mind—is where intelligence exists. This book is intended to help you not only begin with a questioning mind but also return to it continually as you practice, learn, and grow.

When you approach something with an open mind, you are not "thinking" or offering thoughts and opinions. Rather, your mind is empty, ready, and open to the possibilities. Even when you become more proficient, it's important to not adopt the mind of the expert, which is not as open. Instead, enjoy the experience of learning and discovery without an agenda, and without a need to achieve or finish first. Let go of thinking of yourself consciously; when you do so, your practice becomes an expression of your true nature. Through pure effort, your body and mind also become pure. Your practice puts your inner world in order and leads you to the right way of life. You become enlightened.

You truly develop when you look straight into things. By making a genuine effort, instead of simply going through the motions with careless or negligent attempts, you come to know yourself. It is here that you must investigate your inner nature and the connecting principles of all things. You bring light into the darkness. You gain the freedom to act in accordance with your nature, and thus not be deceived by false representations of right and wrong, good or bad. When you understand the nature of the mind, you can no longer be controlled. Nothing outside of yourself will trouble you. You have power and sovereignty.

How to Use This Book

This twelve-week guide is designed to enhance your training through thought, reflection, and application. As I have noted, the book is structured so that it focuses on a specific principle each week. Each day you will read a question that opens the door to your reflections. Take time to think about the question as a meditation before you begin writing. You may do this before or after your practice. You can also spend some time in the early morning, and then review again at the end of your day to add or fine-tune your thoughts. Add the date to your entry. There is enough space for writing so that you can revisit the meditation questions later in the week or even months later. This will enable you to trace your own evolution. The sequence builds on itself, but you are free to jump ahead to a principle that aligns with a particular lesson or epiphany you have experienced.

Remember that in understanding your imperfections, you are gaining self-acceptance and creating a more open and way-seeking mind. You become free of self-judgment and in doing so learn to accept the world as it exists, without meaningless perceptions or preferences. Be sincere and make your way with your best effort in each moment. That is enough. Remember that nirvana is not reached at the end of your training; it exists in the act of the practice itself. In this way, you are no longer restricted or limited.

Before You Begin

Take a few minutes to do a diagnostic check on yourself. Record your response to each question. This will create a baseline from which you can compare your evolution in T'ai Chi.

1. How do you physically feel (loose or stiff, relaxed or tense, heavy or light, for example)?

____

____

____

____

____

2. How are you thinking (fast or slow, positive or negative, etc.)?

____

____

____

____

3. How do you commonly deal with events or
   circumstances?

____

____

____

____

4. How do you deal with other people?

____

____

____

____

5. How can T'ai Chi as a practice help you in some
   or all of these areas?

____

____

____

____

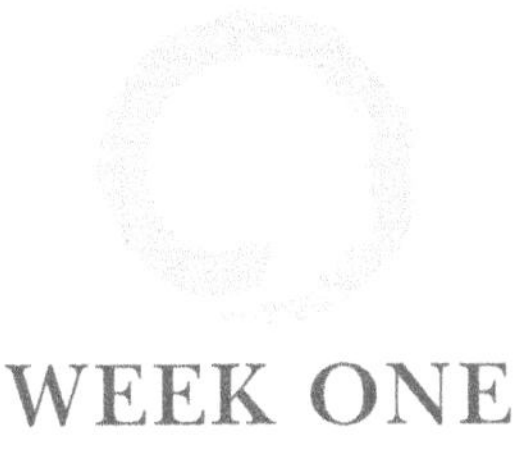

WEEK ONE

Wuji: No Extremes

Before you can learn the T'ai Chi theory of Yin Yang, you must first understand Wuji, which precedes T'ai Chi. According to Wang Zong-Yue's writings, known as the *Taijiquan Classic*:

> [Taiji] is generated from Wuji and is a pivotal function of movement and stillness. It is the mother of Yin and Yang. When it moves, it divides. At rest it reunites.

Westerners can equate Wuji to the state of the universe before the Big Bang. At first there was nothing, and everything was one. The Big Bang was a blast of energy, sending positive and negative charges through the universe. Similarly, the positive and negative forces released from Wuji are the Yin Yang elements: T'ai Chi.

Wuji is a moment of stillness, the state you are in before beginning the T'ai Chi form. Your mind is calm, and your body is in balance with itself. In this state, your mind and body are not divided but unified: oneness and stillness. Once you move, you have entered T'ai Chi.

Wuji is practiced and developed with still meditation.

WHAT HAVE YOU LEARNED ABOUT WUJI IN YOUR T'AI CHI CLASS?

ARE YOU PRESENTLY ABLE TO ATTAIN CALM AND STILLNESS? HOW CAN YOU DEVELOP THIS STATE OF BEING?

____

____

____

____

____

____

____

____

____

____

____

____

HOW DO PHYSICAL STILLNESS AND A CALM MIND INFLUENCE YOUR EMOTIONAL STATE? HOW DO YOU FEEL?

HOW CAN YOU RECOGNIZE WHEN THERE IS AN OPPORTUNITY TO HAVE STILLNESS, EVEN IF ONLY FOR A MOMENT, AND USE THAT OPPORTUNITY TO EXPERIENCE WUJI? WHEN CAN YOU PRACTICE STILL MEDIATION? HOW OFTEN? HOW LONG?

IF WUJI MEANS NO EXTREME OR NO DISCRIMINATION, WHERE CAN YOU SEE THIS AS ONENESS IN THE WORLD?

WHERE DO YOU OBSERVE WUJI (UNDIVIDED) MOVING TO T'AI CHI (YIN YANG) IN YOUR SURROUNDINGS OR IN THE ACTIONS OF EVERYDAY LIFE?

AT THE CLOSE OF YOUR DAY, HOW CAN YOU RETURN TO WUJI, A STATE OF STILLNESS, TO REST?

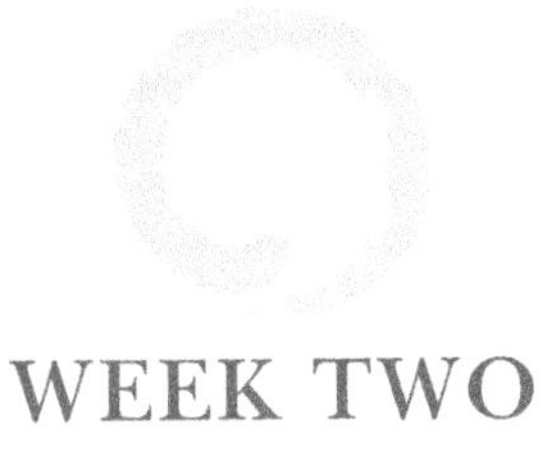

WEEK TWO

Breath

Your breath is the link to the outside world. It is how you interact with and draw energy from the environment around you. The quality of the environment and the quality of your breathing determine the quality of your Qi (energy). Think of it as clean energy.

How you breathe affects your level of energy and your emotional state. Learning to regulate the two through proper breathing can have a lasting impact on your life. It is a vital source of longevity.

Your breathing is also the first step in learning the principles of Yin Yang. If your inhale is Yin, then your exhale is Yang. You cannot have only one. Each must exist for the other. This lesson in the symbiosis of Yin Yang will increasingly reveal itself as you learn and grow in your understanding of T'ai Chi.

WHAT DO YOU NOTICE WHEN YOU FOCUS ON YOUR BREATHING (LENGTH, SMOOTHNESS, DURATION, EVENNESS)?

HOW CAN YOU IMPROVE THE QUALITY OF YOUR BREATHING BEGINNING TODAY?

WHEN CAN YOU FIND TIME IN YOUR DAY TO FOCUS ON QUALITY BREATHING, EVEN FOR TWO MINUTES?

HOW DOES PROPER BREATHING IMPACT YOUR ENERGY? HOW DO YOU FEEL?

WHEN YOUR BREATHING IS CORRECT, HOW DOES IT IMPACT YOUR THINKING?

HOW CAN YOU COORDINATE YOUR BREATHING WITH MOVEMENT, EVEN IN THE SMALLEST TASK?

HOW CAN YOU CARRY FORWARD THIS LESSON ON BREATHING?

WEEK THREE

Learning and Self-Discovery Takes Time

It does not matter how slowly you go,
so long as you do not stop.

—CONFUCIUS

Each week you learn a small detail and in the process are likely to forget the other things you have learned in the class. This is okay! The intention is to take a journey of self-discovery, and this takes time. Each lesson will reinforce what you have learned in other ways and gradually integrate into your practice. The key is to show up, keep at it, and enjoy the unfolding of your new knowledge.

The process of learning begins with attention. In the beginning you are listening intently, observing, and paying attention to minute physical movement. You are also memorizing, and as you may now be aware, there are a lot of details in what appear to be the most casual of movements. This memorization will take time.

Your lessons expose you to the language of T'ai Chi. *Wuji, T'ai Chi, Tao, Wu Wei,* and so many new words and sounds are communicated so that you may explore their meaning. This is another path of conception.

With good instruction and practice, you can organize your new knowledge so that it may be correctly expressed. Expression, even crudely at this stage, completes the cycle of learning, as you are communicating what you know as you understand it at this moment. As a result, your thoughts, emotions, and movements elevate to a higher plane, and you evolve as a human being.

WHAT WAS YOUR EXPERIENCE IN YOUR EARLY T'AI CHI LESSONS? HOW DID YOU FEEL?

WHAT DETAILS DO YOU REMEMBER FROM YOUR LAST LESSON? WHAT ARE YOU LOOKING FOR?

WHAT HAVE YOU PRACTICED MOST FROM YOUR LESSONS? WHAT DO YOU WANT TO PRACTICE MORE?

HAVE YOU CREATED TIME TO PRACTICE EACH DAY, EVEN IF ONLY FOR A SHORT TIME? HOW CAN YOU ENHANCE THIS?

WHEN YOU PRACTICE, HOW DO YOU FEEL DURING THE REST OF YOUR DAY?

HOW CAN DAILY PRACTICE BENEFIT YOU OVER THE LONG TERM?

HOW CAN YOU INVEST IN YOURSELF THROUGH LEARNING AND PRACTICE TO BECOME THE T'AI CHI PRACTITIONER YOU ENVISION YOURSELF TO BE?

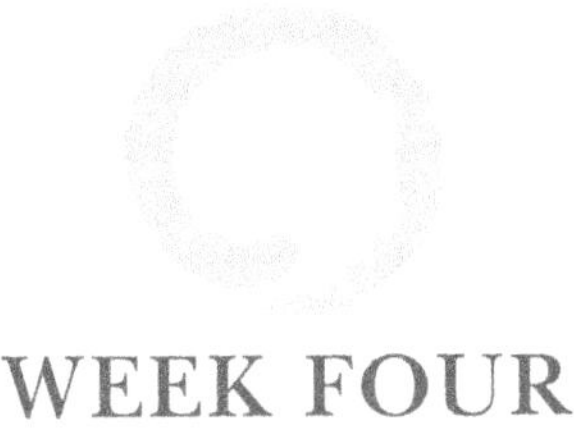

WEEK FOUR

Yin Yang: Integrated Opposites

Everything in nature interacts at some level. This is because the natural world includes all things. There is a connection between stillness and motion, silence and sound, up and down, left and right, forward and backward. Everything is connected, is in motion, and exists in constant transition and change. Nothing remains in a permanent state.

T'ai Chi represents the universal and natural exchange of all things through Yin Yang, the integrated opposites. We cannot have up without down, hot without cold, and even good without bad. Yin Yang exists in the change of seasons, the natural elements (fire and water, for example), and even the relationships we have with each other.

Through this principle you learn that nothing, not even your own thought, is complete without complementary opposition. This awareness brings you to humility and eases your need to seek security in one-sided absolutes or perfection, fixed attitudes, and systems. Instead, you see the reality of life in the wholeness of nature. You gain freedom.

Each movement of T'ai Chi is encoded with Yin Yang, as each contains multiple levels of integrated opposites. It exists in your inhale and exhale, the relative posture of your upper and lower body, the position of your feet, the shifting of weight in your legs, the level of each arm, and the direction of each palm. Every T'ai Chi position expresses Yin Yang in motion. When you move from Yin to Yang, or Yang to Yin, you are training to become relaxed and settled as you experience transition and change without resistance. This training in movement is a physical metaphor for the action of life.

WHERE DID YOU FIND YIN YANG IN THIS WEEK'S T'AI CHI LESSON? OBSERVE AND REFLECT ON THE INTERACTION IN YOUR BREATHING AND MOVEMENT, YOUR STANCES, THE UPPER AND LOWER PARTS OF YOUR BODY, AND THE INTERACTION OF YOUR HANDS.

HOW DO YOU FEEL WHEN YOUR BODY IS CORRECTLY POSITIONED IN YIN YANG FORMS?

HOW DOES MOVING FROM YIN TO YANG, OR FROM YANG TO YIN, IN A SMOOTH, RELAXED WAY IMPACT HOW YOU ARE THINKING?

WHERE DO YOU SEE THE SYMBIOTIC RELATIONSHIP EXPRESSED AS YIN YANG IN YOUR ENVIRONMENT? WHERE DO YOU SEE THE COMPLEMENTARY OPPOSITES? OBSERVE YOUR SURROUNDINGS—THE INTERACTION OF NATURE, YOUR PHYSICAL MOVEMENT, THE INTERACTIONS OF PEOPLE AROUND YOU, PASSIVE AND ACTIVE ELEMENTS, AND SO ON.

HOW CAN YOU APPLY THE YIN YANG CONCEPT OF INTEGRATED OPPOSITES TO SITUATIONS IN YOUR LIFE TODAY?

WHAT HAPPENS WHEN YOU MOVE TOO FAR TO EXTREME YIN OR YANG IN YOUR T'AI CHI OR YOUR LIFE? WHAT CAN YOU DO NEXT?

WHERE CAN YOU FIND A BETTER BALANCE AMONG THE OPPOSITES IN YOUR LIFE?

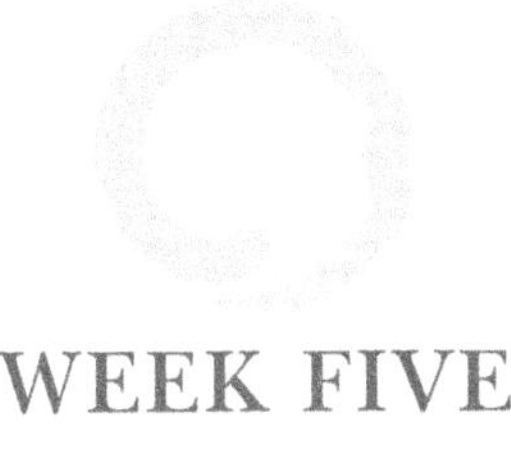

WEEK FIVE

Settle the Qi

Qi Gong and T'ai Chi focus on expanding the lungs to increase your oxygen intake, remove tension from your muscles, and open the joints. Combined, these remove stagnation and allow your circulation to flow unobstructed. This process increases your Qi, or energy, but you do not want to *raise* the Qi.

Every cell in your body contains an electrical charge. The body is composed of approximately 60 percent water, which is an ideal element for conductivity. At your *Dan Tien*, or center of gravity, the combination of muscle, fat, and water creates an ideal environment—a battery to store your Qi.

Settling the Qi is the process that brings your energy to your Dan Tien for storage. This cannot be forced but occurs with awareness. You enter a calm and lucid state, filled with relaxed and flowing energy, as opposed to the frenetic and tension-filled energy that occurs when the Qi is raised into the chest or even the brain.

WHEN PRACTICING THE QI GONG SET(S) YOU HAVE LEARNED, WHERE DO YOU SENSE YOUR QI?

OBSERVE WATER IN THE OCEAN, A BAY, POND, RIVER, OR STREAM. HOW DOES WATER MOVE? HOW IS IT SETTLED, EVEN WHEN MOVING? HOW DOES SETTLING THE QI MIRROR THE CHARACTERISTICS OF WATER?

A RELAXED BODY MEANS SMOOTH, RELAXED MOVEMENT. WHEN YOUR QI IS SETTLED, HOW DOES THIS ENHANCE THE MOVEMENT OF YOUR THOUGHTS? WHAT IS THE EFFECT ON YOUR PHYSICAL ACTIONS?

HOW CAN CULTIVATING THIS SENSE OF SETTLED ENERGY ENHANCE YOUR HEALTH AND WELL-BEING?

HOW CAN YOU MAINTAIN AWARENESS OF SETTLING YOUR QI?

HOW CAN YOU ACCESS THE PRACTICE OF SETTLING YOUR QI EVERY DAY?

WHEN YOU FEEL SETTLED AND YOUR ENERGY IS FLOWING FREELY THROUGH YOUR BODY, YOUR EXPERIENCE OF LIFE BECOMES SOMETHING ELSE. DESCRIBE THIS CHANGE.

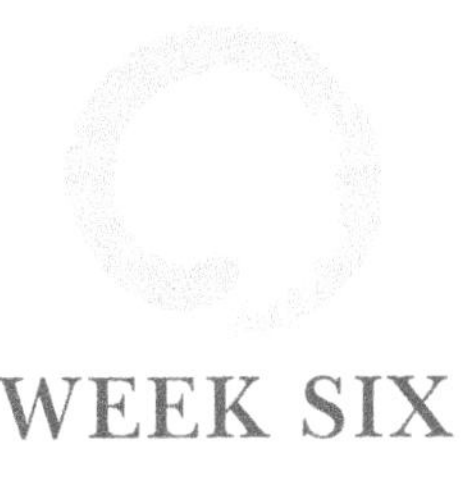

WEEK SIX

Intention

Once you have learned to settle the Qi, next you must learn to use intention to direct its flow. Think of it like this: your *Yi*, or wisdom mind, has access to the energy stored in the Dan Tien, your battery. The mind can draw this energy from the Dan Tien and direct it to any part of the body. Your Qi animates your movement and increases your power in a concentrated way. It is this process that distinguishes T'ai Chi as an internal martial art.

Training intention is accomplished in Qi Gong exercises and T'ai Chi forms. Many beginners start their training with simple breathing sets. The patterns of the arms and hands train the mind to lead the Qi in the direction of the hands: in front of you, out to the sides, up, down, and in circular patterns. Repetition enables your brain to "dial in," making connections within your body by feeling the course of energy.

HOW DOES YOUR CURRENT QI GONG EXERCISE OR T'AI CHI DRILL TRAIN INTENTION?

HOW IS YOUR INTENTION BECOMING MORE FOCUSED?

HOW DO YOU USE INTENTION WHILE REMAINING RELAXED AND SETTLED?

HOW DOES INTENTION BRING YOU INTO THE PRESENT MOMENT?

NOW THAT YOU ARE AWARE THAT INTENTION LEADS YOUR QI, HOW CAN THIS APPLY TO COMMON CHORES OR TASKS YOU DO AT WORK OR AT HOME?

WHAT NON–T'AI CHI ACTIVITIES CAN BE IMPROVED WITH BETTER INTENTION?

WHAT OPPORTUNITIES EXIST FOR YOU TO APPLY YOUR INTENTION AS YOU MOVE THROUGH LIFE?

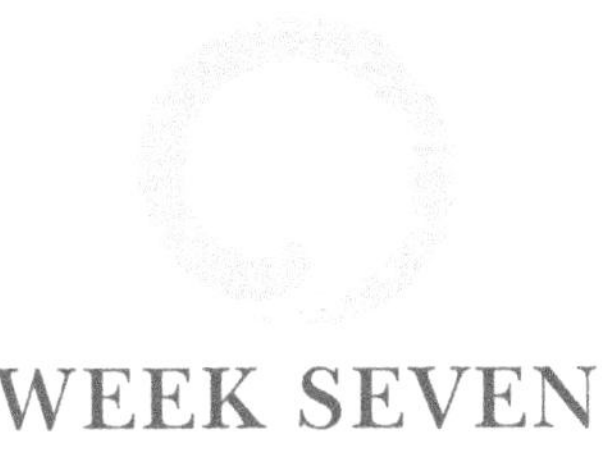

WEEK SEVEN

Your Center

Everything in the world has a center, a focal point or fulcrum, because everything has a center of gravity. It is a recognized element of nature and was a focus in most ancient thinking and writings. This notion remains true in modern times; people still speak of being centered or finding their center. This is because gravity is a sensory signal that has a tremendous impact on the brain's communication with the body. This is especially important to maintain as you age.

Until recently, you may have gone through your life with little or no awareness of your true center of gravity. This is a significant detail, as your center of gravity is the point of balance for your body—where the weight of your body is balanced in all directions. It is also considered a place of understanding. Science is increasingly discovering a second brain, functioning without conscious thought, located at the center, or Dan Tien.

The *Tao de Ching* describes the center as the center of a wheel, from which the spokes emerge to drive the rim into motion. The same applies to the body. While the Yi, or wisdom mind, directs the energy, the Dan Tien steers the body in the intended direction. Every step, twist, turn, kick, block, or strike is directed from the center. This is the center of your mini-universe.

HOW DOES THE MOVEMENT IN YOUR TRAINING REVEAL YOUR CENTER, OR DAN TIEN, TO YOU?

WHAT CAN YOU DO TO IMPROVE YOUR SENSE OF CENTER IN THE TRAINING DRILLS AND FORMS YOU ARE CURRENTLY WORKING ON?

WHEN CAN YOU FIND YOUR CENTER DURING COMMON PHYSICAL MOVEMENT?

HOW DOES WUJI, SETTLING THE QI, AND INTENTION RELATE TO YOUR CENTER?

WHERE DO YOU OBSERVE THE CENTER POINTS ALL AROUND YOU?

HOW CAN YOU FIND A CENTER IN THE ACTIVE OR PASSIVE, FULL OR EMPTY, RESPONSIBILITIES AND PASSIONS OF YOUR LIFE?

WHEN OBSERVING THE INTERPLAY OF LIFE'S EVENTS, HOW CAN YOU CENTER YOURSELF?

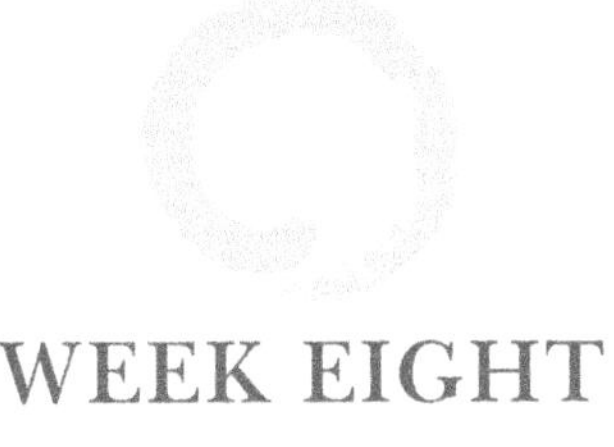

WEEK EIGHT

Rooting

When your body is settled, balanced, and centered, you begin to have good rooting. You establish your roots from the place that touches the ground—the soles of your feet. The contact is firm and continuous.

We see rooting in nature. Observe a tree: its roots are wide and deep, providing a stable base for the branches, which are pliable and able to flex with the wind. We seek to accomplish the same effect in our T'ai Chi.

When you stand with good rooting, your hands, shoulders, elbows, hips, and knees are relaxed. You are not using muscle to fight gravity so that you can remain upright. Doing so expends mental energy, as your Yi must direct the Qi to energize these muscles, which wastes physical energy from the unnecessary physical exertion. With good rooting you do not fight gravity, but instead align with it.

HOW CAN YOU IMPROVE THE SENSE OF ROOTING IN THE T'AI CHI FORMS OR TECHNIQUES YOU ARE LEARNING AND PRACTICING?

HOW DOES YOUR BODY FEEL WHEN YOU HAVE GOOD ROOTING? WHAT DIFFERENCE DO YOU NOTICE WHEN YOU ARE OR ARE NOT ROOTED IN YOUR STANCES?

HOW DOES PROPER ROOTING HELP YOU FEEL RELAXED PHYSICALLY AND MENTALLY?

HOW DOES PROPER ROOTING IMPACT YOUR BALANCE? HOW CAN ROOTING BENEFIT SOMEONE YOU KNOW WITH BALANCE ISSUES?

THE FOLLOWING NON–T'AI CHI ACTIVITIES PRESENT OPPORTUNITIES TO PRACTICE YOUR ROOTING:

IF GOOD ROOTING MEANS HAVING A FIRM FOUNDATION, WHAT OTHER AREAS OF YOUR LIFE COULD BENEFIT FROM HAVING STRONGER ROOTING?

MEDITATION CAN BE A FORM OF ROOTING, IN THAT . . .

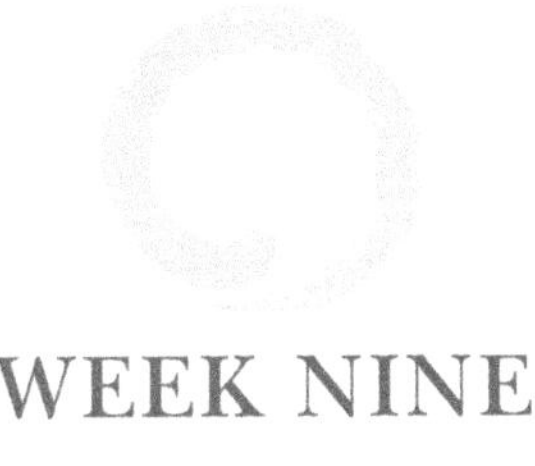

WEEK NINE

Alignment

Proper body alignment is an essential component for good T'ai Chi—and for good health. Alignment from head to toe reduces stress on the body while increasing power and efficiency. Proper alignment enhances your rooting and creates a clear path of energy through each part of your form, which increases your ability to issue power.

Proper body alignment decreases wear and tear on the joints. It reduces neck, back, shoulder, and knee pain. It also reduces muscle aches and fatigue because the joints are no longer being used to compensate for poor alignment. Some reports suggest that proper body alignment enhances the functioning of the digestive, respiratory, and nervous systems, too.

Simple awareness of and subtle adjustments for correct alignment will improve your T'ai Chi and can have a profound impact on your total health and sense of well-being.

OBSERVE WHEN YOU MOVE IN THE T'AI CHI OR QI GONG SETS, OR IN COMMON MOVEMENT. NOTICE YOUR ALIGNMENT AND LOOK FOR MINOR ACHES OR FEELINGS OF RESISTANCE. RECORD WHAT YOU FEEL.

DESCRIBE A T'AI CHI FORM YOU ARE WORKING ON, AND IDENTIFY WHERE THERE ARE OPPORTUNITIES FOR BETTER ALIGNMENT.

HOW IS PROPER BODY ALIGNMENT CHANGING YOUR PHYSIOLOGY? WHAT ARE THE MENTAL AND PSYCHOLOGICAL CHANGES YOU ARE EXPERIENCING?

WHAT COMMON MOVEMENTS ARE IMPROVING WITH BETTER BODY ALIGNMENT?

COMPARE YOUR LEVEL OF ENERGY BEFORE AND AFTER EXPERIENCING PROPER BODY ALIGNMENT.

OBSERVE THE ENVIRONMENT AROUND YOU. RECORD STRUCTURES THAT ARE ALIGNED WELL AND CONSIDER THE IMPACT OF POOR ALIGNMENT.

ALIGNMENT IS A PHYSICAL TRAIT BUT CAN EXIST SITUATIONALLY, TOO. HOW DOES ALIGNING WITH A CURRENT SITUATION REDUCE RESISTANCE AND STRESS WHILE BENEFITING YOU AND YOUR OVERALL WELL-BEING?

WEEK TEN

Meditation + Qi Gong = T'ai Chi

At some point in training, your meditation and Qi Gong sets begin to progress into the basic forms and techniques of T'ai Chi. This progression follows the historical development of this martial art. The earliest practitioners knew that one's overall health is dependent on a healthy mind, which was accomplished through meditation. Next came physical Qi Gong sets to improve health for the body. It was only later that martial artists realized how the system could also generate power and incorporated T'ai Chi training concepts into their system of fighting. T'ai Chi ("grand ultimate") became T'ai Chi Chuan ("grand ultimate fist"). When you train in this progression, you are reliving centuries of history over the course of weeks and months.

As you begin to learn T'ai Chi forms, be mindful of their roots—meditation and Qi Gong—and always include them in your training.

HOW HAS MEDITATION BECOME A PART OF YOUR LIFE PRACTICE?

DESCRIBE HOW QI GONG SETS ARE CHANGING THE WAY YOU FEEL, YOUR ENERGY LEVEL, AND THE WAY YOU MOVE.

HOW ARE MEDITATION AND QI GONG INFLUENCING YOUR T'AI CHI?

DESCRIBE HOW MEDITATION AND QI GONG INFORM AND SUPPORT YOUR T'AI CHI AND PRODUCE THE SENSATION OF A RISE IN POWER.

HOW IS PRACTICING DAILY MEDITATION, QI GONG, AND T'AI CHI INFLUENCING YOUR SENSE OF WELL-BEING AND A LUCID, BALANCED STATE OF MIND? HOW CAN YOU SUSTAIN THIS STATE OF BEING THROUGHOUT THE DAY, EVERY DAY?

HOW DOES DEVELOPING THIS INTERNAL POWER MAKE YOU FEEL EMPOWERED IN YOUR LIFE?

WHAT IS YOUR TRAINING GOAL MOVING FORWARD?

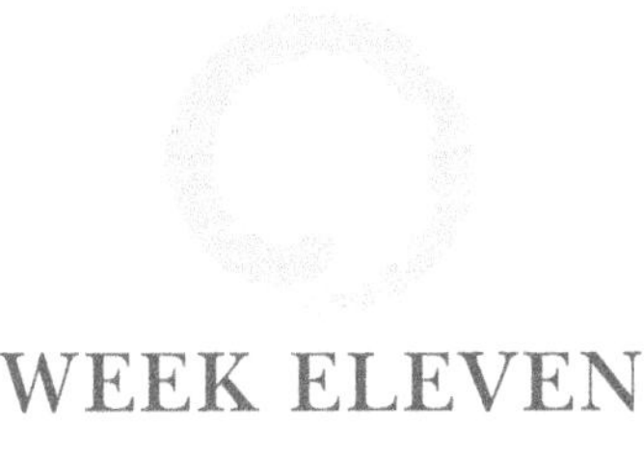

WEEK ELEVEN

Principle or Sequence—
Where Is the Focus?

You may not be aware how much you have learned in these early weeks of training. As you might have realized, some techniques or exercises seem simple, but there is a right way to do them. If you can internalize these core concepts early in your training, you are beginning a life of T'ai Chi with a strong foundation. It is in mastering these subtleties that you achieve the art.

The trick here is to maintain a focus on the fundamentals. It is quite common to want to focus on the *sequence* of movements as opposed to concentrating on the technique itself.

Focusing on the sequence only means moving in the right order, however. It is not as valuable as doing the set with proper alignment, breathing, and intention, for example. To illustrate the point, consider the difference in meaning between these two phrases: 1) doing the right things, and 2) doing things right. One is effective, while the other is efficient. Ideally, you want both, but one must be in place before the other can add value.

When training the T'ai Chi form, learn the sequence, but focus on the principles. The sequence will always come. Then your T'ai Chi will look and feel more complete.

WHAT DETAILS HAVE YOU FOCUSED ON IN TRAINING AND PRACTICE? WHERE HAVE YOU SEEN IMPROVEMENT?

WHAT CAN YOU FOCUS ON TO INCREASE THE QUALITY OF YOUR T'AI CHI? HOW CAN YOU DO THIS?

WHAT PRINCIPLE OF T'AI CHI WOULD YOU LIKE TO LEARN MORE ABOUT? WHY?

HOW CAN IMPROVING ONE ELEMENT OF YOUR T'AI CHI TRAINING BENEFIT OTHER PARTS OF YOUR PRACTICE?

DESCRIBE THE DIFFERENCE IN FEELING WHEN YOU ARE AND ARE NOT PERFORMING THE T'AI CHI FORM OR A QI GONG SEQUENCE WITH RELAXED INTENTION, ROOTING, BALANCE, AND ALIGNMENT.

WHEN LEARNING SOMETHING NEW OR TRAINING FOR A NEW TASK IN YOUR WORK, DO YOU FOCUS ON LEARNING THE PRINCIPLES BEFORE THE SEQUENCE OR PROCESS? HOW DOES THIS IMPACT YOUR ABILITY TO USE THE KNOWLEDGE WITH CONSISTENCY AND QUALITY?

HOW DO YOU SPEND YOUR DAY ON COMMON ACTIVITIES? ARE YOU PRESENT OR GOING THROUGH THE MOTIONS? ARE YOU ACTIVELY PARTICIPATING IN YOUR LIFE OR SLEEPWALKING THROUGH IT? HOW CAN YOU BE MORE AWARE OF THE QUALITY OF THE MOMENT WITHIN THE SEQUENCE OF EVENTS THAT UNFOLD IN YOUR DAY (DOING HOUSEWORK, SPENDING TIME WITH FAMILY, PERFORMING YOUR JOB, COOKING, READING, AND SO ON)?

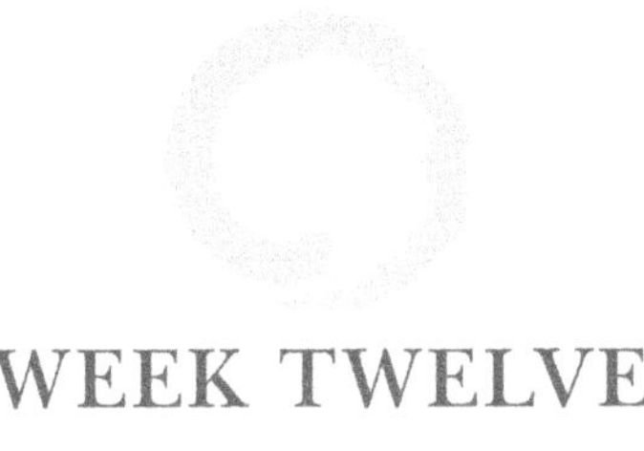

WEEK TWELVE

Your T'ai Chi Path

Many people begin T'ai Chi with a certain perception, only to find that what they originally perceived was just the tip of the iceberg. T'ai Chi reveals itself gradually over time. Through practice and study, you come to an awareness of the meaning of T'ai Chi: the grand ultimate. By choosing to begin training in T'ai Chi, you have discovered a passage to a way of living that is natural, vast, and ever unfolding.

You begin to align with universal laws. You develop endurance and resilience. You become more flexible in body and mind. You are training yourself in a way that can last a lifetime.

You must continue to grow and refine yourself. You must continue to reflect on how the universal principles apply to your Qi Gong, T'ai Chi, and everyday life. You must bring the practice out of the classroom and into your daily way of living. In doing so, you can achieve something beyond learning a martial art: a lifetime of self-cultivation.

AS YOU REFLECT ON THESE TWELVE WEEKS OF TRAINING, WHAT HAVE YOU LEARNED?

DESCRIBE THE CHANGES THAT MEDITATION, QI GONG, AND T'AI CHI HAVE INFLUENCED IN YOUR LIFE.

HOW HAS TRAINING IN T'AI CHI ALTERED YOUR PERCEPTION AND PERSPECTIVE?

HOW HAVE YOUR THOUGHTS AND FEELINGS EVOLVED OVER THE LAST TWELVE WEEKS?

HOW HAS YOUR OVERALL SENSE OF WELL-BEING CHANGED SINCE TRAINING IN T'AI CHI?

HOW HAS YOUR TRAINING IMPACTED YOUR THOUGHTS ABOUT LIFE AND THE MEANING OF YOUR LIFE?

AS YOU LOOK FORWARD TO YOUR LIFE AS A T'AI CHI PRACTITIONER, THE VISION OF YOURSELF IS:

BONUS QUESTION: MOVING FORWARD IN YOUR T'AI CHI TRAINING, YOU RESOLVE TO . . .

FINAL THOUGHTS

This book is intended as a beginning guide to a lifetime of self-cultivation. The end of this book should not be the end of your process of self-discovery, self-reflection, self-cultivation, and self-refinement. In fact, it is my hope that this is your *starting* point.

I leave you with a few ideas for assistance and encouragement as you continue your path on a life of T'ai Chi:

- Review the diagnostic questions at the beginning of the book. Make note of the changes and what you want to continue to develop. Create a new diagnostic today and set a calendar date in six and twelve months to review and compare.

- If this book has promoted discussions with your Sifu (instructor) or other students, then continue to keep those channels of communication open. We can learn a lot from each other.

- Remember to maintain the open-minded approach of a beginner. This enables you to continue to grow. To me, an open mind is the true fountain of youth.

- You may be making discoveries and progressing in leaps and bounds, but eventually the progress becomes more subtle. Do not be discouraged, and do not allow yourself to plateau.

- Persistence, practice, and patience are greater assets than natural talent. Remain disciplined in your approach, and you will become a T'ai Chi master in your own time.

- There are many other sources of information, and there are many perspectives on this martial art. Invest the time to go further into the traditional writings of the *Tao de Ching*, the T'ai Chi classics, and other books to learn the deeper meaning of T'ai Chi. Continue to explore, learn, and incorporate what feels good and is useful for you.

- Over time and with practice, you'll find your own unique way of expressing T'ai Chi. This is the *art* of martial arts. Be yourself.

ACKNOWLEDGMENTS

When I stop to consider how many people spark a thought, action, idea, or direction for me on any given day, the number is staggering. Still, there are those who are in closer proximity and offer themselves directly with suggestions, advice, and encouragement. To all of them, named and unnamed, I am forever grateful.

I would like to thank Billie Fitzpatrick for continued guidance, and Maureen Forys and Rachel Monaghan at Happenstance for the thought, care, and energy you give to create something special and unique. I am glad I met all of you.

To Sifu Gus Kaparos, Boris Gluzberg, Greg Brower, Mark Schnurman, Darlene Famiglietti, and Violet Li: thanks for your support and allowing me to think out loud.

My students are each unique in their aspirations and abilities. Each of you presents an opportunity to bring the art of T'ai Chi alive in a way that is singular. Your questions, enthusiasm, commitment, and striving help keep this art alive—and influenced this book.

And of course, Jeanne and Shannon, for always reminding me of what is most important.

ABOUT THE AUTHOR

William Donnelly has made an art of his life. He is a musician and composer, author, martial artist, entrepreneur, career expert, and teacher. Bill has been practicing T'ai Chi Chuan for over twenty-five years. He teaches the philosophical, health, and martial elements of the art, which he studied and developed in addition to Kung Fu at the Green Cloud Martial Arts Academy in New York.

Bill has been invited to workshops and speaking engagements and is a frequent demonstrator at World T'ai Chi Day events. He continues to teach T'ai Chi's traditional applications, in addition to applications for conflict resolution, life, and business strategies, in group or private sessions for corporations, executives, entrepreneurs, and individuals.

He is the author of *Inner Secrets: Discovering T'ai Chi's Hidden Lessons for Preservation, Protection, and Peace of Mind*, available from Amazon.com, Barnes & Noble, and other online retailers.

For private instruction, appearances, or speaking engagements, visit *www.privatetaichi.net*.